LOST IN HEALTH

LOST IN HEALTH

Lori Lynn Paul

ISBN: 1514876930
Softcover ISBN-13: 9781514876930

Printed in the United States of America

First Printing:

CreateSpace.com

www.powerup2health.com

This book is dedicated to my daughters, Ella and Brityn, who inspire me every day with their infectious smiles and tender hearts.

Table of Contents

Introduction ·ix

Chapter 1 My Unexpected Journey· · · · · · · · · · · · · · · · · · · 1

Chapter 2 Writing the Ship· 8

Chapter 3 Juiced Up· 13

Chapter 4 Finding Myself· 20

Chapter 5 Cleansed Mind· 26

Chapter 6 All About Me · 31

Chapter 7 Gratitude for Love · 37

Chapter 8 Broken Home· 42

Chapter 9 Gotta Have Faith · 50

Chapter 10 Love or Money· 54

Chapter 11 All Powered Up · 57

Introduction

To those I may have wronged, I ask forgiveness. To those I may have helped,
I wish I did more. To those I neglected to help, I ask for understanding.
To those who helped me, I sincerely thank you very much.

—DAVID AVOCADO WOLFE

My health journey started when I least expected it. I guess they all do, don't they? It came out of the blue and slapped me in the face. Without knowing where my journey would lead, without knowing what decisions were ahead, without knowing what the outcome would be, I innocently forged ahead. One positive aspect of my health journey was and still is the amazing people in my life. I was not aware of how wonderful they were until I went through many rounds of health issues, but in the end, I learned the meaning of true friendship and unconditional love.

First, I want to thank my father. Thank you for being a listening ear, a supportive arm, and a never-ending love for my bad moods or complaining. Dad, your weekly check-ins and true concern for my health were and still are so much appreciated. Knowing how much you cared made me see I was not alone.

Second, thank you to my husband, Christian. Christian, you showed me true devotion through sickness and in health. You grabbed and hung onto the marriage vows when I did not and stayed by my side when I was struggling the most. Christian, you were my guardian angel and lifted me up when I was at my lowest. Thank you from the bottom of my heart!

Third, thank you to a couple very dear friends. Thank you for sticking with me through tough decisions, through not making the best choices, and even through some good decisions. (Yes, I made some!) Your constant empathy and lack of judgment made my journey bearable, livable, and ultimately successful!

Dad, Christian, and my dear friends, all of your continuous love, caring nature, and compassion helped me learn and understand the true meaning of love and friendship. And mostly, you all allowed me to get back up on my two feet when I did not think I could stand. Thank you all for being willing to break through my armor, walking beside me, always loving me, allowing me to fail, yet always reassuring me I was not on this journey alone. Words cannot express how much your unconditional love, friendship, and support led me through the dark days. With all of my love and appreciation…thank you.

My Unexpected Journey

Never give up. Great things take time.

—WISE MAN SI

Waking up from an emergency surgery with my husband standing over my bed saying, "Lori, do you know what happened? You had a hole in your bladder!" *What? How is this possible?* Earlier that evening, after having dinner with my mom, who was staying with us for the Memorial Day weekend in 2012, I began to feel some pain in my abdomen. The pain was not cramping or a stomachache, just achy. Around ten o'clock that night, I started having more severe pain. I had recently had a procedure done, so I thought maybe this was related. I called the nurse's line to explain my symptoms, but they reassured me this pain was completely unrelated. When I tried to rest, I found the pain was becoming sharper, more constant, and more severe. The pain got to a point where I could not stand upright. I could only sit hunched over on my bed. Finally, at one o'clock in the morning, I asked my husband to take me to the ER. It was a blessing my mother was there, so we did not have to try to find someone to come to the house to stay with our young daughters.

Well, the first trip to the ER was uneventful. They gave me pain relief medication and monitored my vitals. After about three hours, they sent me home. The following morning around eleven o'clock, I could not tolerate the pain again, even with heavy pain medication, so we made a second trip to the ER. This time, they decided to do a little investigation. They performed a CT scan, an MRI, and numerous blood tests. All the test results showed nothing! *Really? Something was going on!* As the pain continued to increase, the ER doctor suggested they call my ob-gyn. Shortly after the call, they transported me by ambulance to another hospital, where my doctor met us. After an examination, my doctor suggested the pain may be caused by a twisted ovary. *What? A twisted ovary?*

To give this surgery more perspective, let's rewind to a year and a half earlier to November 2010, when I was thirty-four years old. I had a partial hysterectomy. Thankfully, they were able to retain my cervix and ovaries because I wanted to keep my ovaries in the rare case we wanted to try for a third child through surrogacy. The reason for the hysterectomy was because my ob-gyn suspected I had adenomyosis. My doctor explained adenomyosis is basically endometriosis on the inside of the uterus instead of the outside. I had been experiencing heavy and excessive periods often times lasting two weeks, painful intercourse (it felt like razor blades), and severe cramping. After the hysterectomy, my doctor confirmed I had severe adenomyosis and said my uterus was so flabby and full of disease it was a blessing they removed it.

Immediately after my hysterectomy, I made massive changes to my lifestyle and my diet. I started eating healthier by cutting out sweets and processed foods. I added protein shakes and ate lean meats like chicken and turkey instead of burgers and steaks. I eliminated alcohol during the week and began to exercise on a daily basis. I started lifting weights, running, and biking versus just walking. Through these changes, I eventually lost nearly twenty pounds, dropped several pant sizes, and was feeling better, fitter, and leaner than I had my entire life.

Fast-forward eighteen months from my hysterectomy to my current surgery. My doctor, knowing my history, was concerned I could lose my ovary if it was twisted. He highly recommended he go in with a scope to view what was happening in my abdomen. After much reluctance, I agreed. The next thing I remember was waking up from the emergency surgery with my husband standing over my bed saying, "Lori, do you know what happened? You had a hole in your bladder." *What? I'm healthier than I've ever been. How could this happen?*

After getting past the shock and surprise, I found out when my doctor went in with the scope that there was urine in my abdomen. The negative results from the CT scan, MRI, and blood tests now made sense. Urine is sterile, so it does not cause vomiting, and it does not show as a foreign substance on the scans, blood tests, or x-rays. Upon finding the urine, my ob-gyn immediately called a urologist to have my bladder repaired. They took biopsies as well, and my ob-gyn said they found endometriosis on my bladder. My doctor believed the endometriosis penetrated my bladder, causing my bladder to rupture. Yes, this was the start of my health journey—one I never thought I would encounter!

Recovering from this surgery was challenging, to say the least. I had to endure a catheter for two weeks following the surgery. Yes, I had to carry a pee bag with me 24-7 for two solid weeks—an experience I hope to have only once in my lifetime! After a week with the catheter, I thought it would be removed; however, the urologist said I had to wait at least one more week due to the extent of the rupture. *Major tears! Major disappointment!* To top things off, shortly thereafter, I developed a urinary tract infection. *Now I have a pee bag for one more week and a painful infection. Could it get any worse?* I survived the additional week with the catheter and the infection. I had another procedure to ensure my bladder was healed and celebrated when they removed the catheter. I truly thought this would have been the end of my journey. Unfortunately, it was only the beginning.

My doctor wanted to treat the endometriosis very aggressively because the endometriosis had grown so severe that it now had penetrated my bladder within eighteen months of my hysterectomy. The first treatment was surgery to remove the remaining endometriosis, then medicine to kill the microscopic cells, and, finally, long-term medicine to keep the endometriosis at bay. I most certainly did not want to experience anything like a ruptured bladder again, so I agreed to the aggressive treatment.

Within six months of my bladder surgery, I had a laparoscopic surgery to remove the remaining endometriosis. My ob-gyn recommended I then start Depro Lupron (a shot once per month for six months) to kill the microscopic cells of endometriosis.[1] My doctor explained the medicine would trigger my body to stop producing hormones, effectively putting my body into menopause. I started the shot within a month after my laparoscopic surgery. The first couple months of taking the shot were fine, but the last several months were not. I ended up suffering from severe fatigue, tired muscles, night sweats, acne, weight gain, and mild hot flashes. *Oh joy!* I finished the shot. It

---

1 http://womenshealth.about.com/cs/hormones/a/lupron.htm

was not easy. Then my ob-gyn recommended I take birth control to maintain what now should be an endometriosis-free body. Still trying to recover from the Lupron shot, I reluctantly agreed. Unfortunately, the birth-control dosage was so robust that I suffered severe depression within two weeks of taking it. My doctor changed my dosage and said we may need to experiment with different doses and brands before we found one that worked.

In light of all of this, my ob-gyn suggested I also see an endocrinologist to have my thyroid checked due to symptoms I was experiencing. Within a week of going to an endocrinologist, the blood-test results showed I had slight hyperthyroidism (overfunctioning thyroid).[2] The endocrinologist did not think it was severe enough to treat, so he told me to come back in six months to have my blood tested again. That was good news—or so I thought at the time!

It was now a year following my bladder surgery and a few months following the Lupron shot, and I was still managing the birth control medication, yet I was not feeling well. I was feeling severely run-down, experienced frequent UTIs, had severe pressure in my bladder, and had frequent urination day and night. To make matters worse, the pain during intercourse had returned. Yes, this had been a problem before, but this severe pain was starting to cause marital issues. The lack of intimacy was bound to take its toll. As a result of all of the symptoms,

---

2 https://en.wikipedia.org/wiki/Hyperthyroidism

I went back to visit my ob-gyn. After a few tests and examinations, my ob-gyn said I had interstitial cystitis. With this new disease, he recommended I take an additional prescription for six to twelve months, have weekly bladder installations (in which the bladder is filled with medication via a catheter for a few seconds up to twenty minutes before being drained or voided),[3] try vaginal valium suppositories (insertion of valium into the vagina to loosen the muscles), and start pelvic floor therapy. *Seriously? More drugs? More appointments? More treatment?* And the journey continued...

---

3 http://www.ic-network.com/conditions/interstitial-cystitis/exploring-treatments/bladder-instillations/

2

Writing the Ship

*Remember that missteps and mistakes are inevitable and you'll
never catch a wave without getting wet.*

—BEGIN WITH YES

Now I was managing more drugs (prescription for endometriosis, bladder infections, and interstitial cystitis) and more doctor
appointments (ob-gyn, endocrinologist, and pelvic-floor therapy) and
feeling worse. To make matters worse in September 2013, I also visited
a family doctor for a health-insurance screening and was diagnosed
with central hypothyroidism. The family doctor referred me to yet
another endocrinologist to confirm the results. This new finding was
surprising because if you remember a year prior, I had been diagnosed
with hyperthyroidism (overfunctioning thyroid). Now, my blood tests
showed central hypothyroidism (thyroid disfunction due to a disorder

of the pituitary gland).[4] To add to the increasing diagnoses, the trips to the new endocrinologist led to being tested and ultimately diagnosed with thyroiditis and two autoimmune diseases: Graves' disease and Hashimoto's disease. *OK, I give up!*

Throughout the past year and a half of receiving more diagnoses and more drugs and seeing more doctors and specialists, I was becoming frustrated, sad, and angry. I was starting to feel that every time I would see a new doctor, I received a new, often different, diagnosis. I was given new drugs to deal with the new diagnosis, which often led to more drugs to help reduce the side effects of the new drugs. At one point, I was taking sixteen medications and supplements daily. Funny thing…I was prescribed four additional drugs I did not even take. *Ugh!* I needed to find an outlet, and fast! My frustrations were building. I was becoming more upset with doctors, with people, and with my health.

My saving grace was that I had heard about journaling from various practitioners. I was told journaling would be a great way to get my frustrations, fears, sadness, anger, and daily thoughts out of my head. Journaling was an outlet for my emotions instead of keeping them all building up inside. Having never kept a journal before, I did not have a clue where to start. So, with my built-up frustration, I started by writing notes to people I was upset with to identify the feelings and

---

4 http://pituitarydisorder.net/central_hypothyroidism.html

emotions I was experiencing. I had no intentions of sending the notes; I just thought it would be very therapeutic to write them. Writing was supposed to help mitigate my frustrations, my sadness, and my emotions. And it did! After feeling so much better after writing the notes, I purchased a notebook and tried to find five to ten minutes every day or every other day to write. I generally wrote in the evenings after the kids went to bed since this was the only time I could find a quiet spot in the house. I began to write my thoughts from the day: the bad things that happened and the good things that happened, whether it was about the office, home, kids, spouse, or friends.

As I continued to journal, I found it very healing to put everything on paper and let it sit there instead of inside of me. My frustrations with my health would fester the longer I held it in, so by writing something and knowing no one would see or read it, it allowed me to let go of the anger, the frustration, and the sadness I felt. As I continued my journaling, I found myself writing a few minutes a couple times a week or five minutes every day. I even had days I would write for thirty to forty-five minutes. I had lots to say!

After telling a friend about my story, she mentioned I should start my own blog if I was comfortable and willing to share my health journey publicly. I was not open to the idea of sharing my story, my thoughts, or my health journey with anyone outside of whom I chose. Writing a blog was scary and so public! I was a very private person. Many friends did not know about my ongoing health issues, and I certainly did not want to share my problems with strangers. Yikes! Despite my concern, my friend and my husband continued to push me, saying a blog would be a great way to share my story or at least document my journey.

As I began to consider the idea, I spent much time weighing the pros and cons and trying to decide if I was ready to expose my health journey to the world. I eventually asked a coworker who had created his own blog for advice on how to start a blog. He suggested I use WordPress.com (WordPress) and said I had to first determine a name for the blog. *A name for my blog? Who knew I would have to name my blog?* Shortly thereafter, I was sitting in a continuing legal-education class when I decided to brainstorm names for a potential blog. I wrote at least fifty potential names. After coming up with so many names, I was so excited and decided right then that I could do this. I was going to write my own blog. I began researching available URLs and eventually narrowed down the name options. Jeez, this had dramatically reduced my name selection because of the availability of names.

After researching a few available URLs, I settled on www. PowerUp2Health.com. I used WordPress for my host due to the low costs and easy formatting. WordPress was exactly what I needed as a newbie at blogging. I chose to begin writing about my childhood health history. I made my first entries very brief and provided a time-line up to the current date. When I finished my childhood history and arrived at the current date, I knew it was time to go live. OMG! My heart was pounding, my hands were sweating, and I felt I was going to have a heart attack. Could I really go public with all of this personal information? What would my friends and my family say?

A couple days later, I went live! *OMG! What did I just do?* I had never felt so nervous yet empowered in my whole life. My story was out there for the world to see. After feeling like I was going to have a nervous breakdown because of all the mixed emotions, I settled into the idea and began to add updates to my blog as I went to new doctors and received new diagnoses. I wanted to keep the blog funny and lighthearted so people could see the happy Lori, not the sad, frustrated Lori. I eventually discovered that writing the blog was my time to think and brainstorm. It was an opportunity to bring others into my struggle and hopefully gain followers who were also struggling with the same or similar problems. I was actually hoping my blog would open other doors for suggestions and referrals for recovery. I was loving it!

3

Juiced Up

Don't worry about doing it right, just get started.

—Unknown

Journaling was a great start to my new health journey regimen. I was still struggling with frustration, sadness, and a "why me" attitude, but I was finding I could manage my emotions more easily through journaling. One day, when speaking to another friend, she introduced me to her neighbor. As the neighbor and I talked, we eventually fell upon the subject of my health. She immediately recommended I visit a friend of hers who was a naturopath. I really had never been much into the idea of nontraditional medicine. However, with my continuing problems and long list of treatments and medications, I thought maybe a more holistic approach could give me greater insight. Honestly, I was a bit hesitant. I really did have faith the traditional doctors knew more than holistic practitioners, but what the heck—it was only a couple hours out of my day.

Making an appointment relatively quickly, I initially met with the naturopath for about two hours. She asked many questions about my childhood and my current history as well as my family history of illness, cancer, and disease. After much discussion, her consensus was that I had liver dysfunction because I was suffering from severe bloating, cracking fingernails, food allergies, autoimmune problems, and dry skin and hair, to just name a few symptoms. The naturopath recommended I complete a twenty-one-day liver cleanse. I was willing to try it but had a winter vacation planned in January 2014, so told her I would start after I returned from vacation. I went on vacation and returned feeling more bloated and fatigued then I had in months. As soon as I started the twenty-one-day cleanse, I began to feel better. After twenty-one days, I felt amazing and lost some weight even though I was not able to exercise because I had sprained my back at the gym. This was great—I did not realize how changing my diet could impact my weight and my health so much. I was feeling better, yet I was beginning to suffer again from severe fatigue and bloating, and now my hands and feet were swelling at different times in the day.

I contacted the naturopath to explain my new symptoms, and she suggested perhaps I had dysbiosis. Dysbiosis is a condition caused by a disruption to the natural flora that inhabits our bowels.[5] A common cause is from use of antibiotics.[6] I had had my share of antibiotics, and now with cleansing my body, my gut flora was out of balance. While this was good news, I did not bother to ask for treatment because I was so upset with how my gut flora could be out of balance when I had just completed a liver cleanse. *Seriously? I think the naturopath is making stuff up!* What this news did trigger was some research, and it became apparent I likely did have dysbiosis; resulting in my body not absorbing the nutrients from the food I was eating. Basically, the nutrients, water, and minerals were going into my body but staying on the outside of my organs and cells instead of being absorbed and used within my body. The research suggested my current illnesses, especially the various autoimmune diseases, could block the absorption of nutrients.[7] Guess what the symptoms were? Yep—fatigue, bloating, and swelling of the hands and feet. The question became, if my body was not absorbing nutrients through healthy food intake, what was I supposed to eat? Ah, the wonderful benefits of juice! I learned that by drinking fresh juice made from fruits and vegetables, my body could rapidly absorb

5 http://www.fernlifecenter.com/imbalances-of-the-gut-flora-in-the-gi-tract%E2%80%A6or-dysbiosis/

6 http://www.fernlifecenter.com/imbalances-of-the-gut-flora-in-the-gi-tract%E2%80%A6or-dysbiosis/

7 http://www.puristat.com/malabsorption/default.aspx

more nutrients.[8] For instance, my body may absorb 90 percent of nutrients from fresh juices, whereas it may only be able to absorb 20 percent of the nutrients from the food I was eating.

I did not have much energy to change my diet and certainly did not know anything about juice options other than orange, apple, and cranberry. As I have learned, those juices are not necessarily the healthiest options on the market, especially if not consumed in moderation. Yet, because my symptoms, like fatigue, bloating, and swelling of my hands and feet were becoming more severe, I made the decision to look at my options for juicing. Without expending too much time and effort, I found a juice company online called Pressed Juicery[9] and purchased a three-day juice cleanse. This company would ship six fresh juices per day for as many as seven days directly to my door. They labeled the bottles for ease of which to drink first, second, third, etc. Hallelujah! I could not imagine drinking only juice for one, three, or seven days, but I also did not have to go grocery shopping, make a meal plan, or cook. And if it made me feel better—bonus!

Having completed the three-day juice cleanse, I was feeling better. I actually liked juicing so much, I bought a used juicer from a neighbor. I started experimenting with oranges for orange juice, and

---

8 http://www.living-foods.com/articles/benefits.html
9 www.Pressedjuicery.com

then thought, *Why not look at the ingredients from various juices and try making my own vegetable juice?* Juicing only vegetables like kale, spinach, celery, and cucumber was very bland. I did get a helpful hint to remove the stem from the kale to reduce the bitterness! That was a lifesaver. In addition, I found that by adding small amounts of fruit, the juice would be sweeter; the fruit helped cover up the bitterness of the greens. I would often add a few pieces of apple or for more sweetness, a few pieces of pineapple. Delicious! As I became more experienced and started to enjoy the juice, I started to reduce the amount of fruit and just focused on the greens.

By juicing, I found I had more energy; my skin, hair, and nails were starting to look healthier; and I was able to reduce my estrogen and allergy medications and remove my thyroid supplement. The bloating was reduced, and I did not experience swelling of my hands and feet again. And to top it off, juicing was a simple and easy way to get my daily fruit and veggie servings. By adding eight ounces of fresh, cold-pressed juice every day, my health seemed to be improving, and my symptoms were reduced substantially.

My go-to juice is all greens, but I do add a piece of fruit now and then when my sweet tooth is acting up. I do not miss a day without my juice. And, because I love juicing so much, here are a couple of my favorite recipes. Remember, you can add a whole apple or cup of pine-apple to any of the below recipes for a much sweeter taste.

GO GREEN

3 cups kale (stem removed)

2 cups spinach

1 cup romaine

1 cup celery

2 small cucumbers

Couple leaves of parsley

Half lemon

½ tbsp. ginger

Dash of cayenne pepper

JUST BEET IT

2 cups kale (stem removed)

2 cups spinach

1 cup romaine

1 cup celery

2 small cucumbers

½ beet (cooked)

Couple leaves of parsley

¼ lemon

1 tbsp. ginger

APPLE A DAY

2 cups kale (stem removed)

2 cups spinach

1 cup romaine

1 apple

1 cup celery

2 small cucumbers

Couple leaves of parsley

¼ lemon

1 tbsp. ginger

4

Finding Myself

Forget all the reasons it won't work, and believe the one reason it will.

—Unknown

Having now seen the benefits of juicing, I was on a roll with getting my health back to normal. The problem was that I still was not feeling 100 percent yet, and I was dealing with the multiple diagnoses of endometriosis, hyperthyroidism, thyroiditis, central hypothyroidism, interstitial cystitis, Graves' disease, Hashimoto's disease, liver dysfunction, and dysbiosis. I felt like I was on a roller coaster. I would try a new treatment, feel better, and then inevitably start to experience new symptoms, or the old symptoms would return. This in turn led me to seek more doctors and receive more suggested treatments. *Up, down, up, down!*

I did not want to admit it, but I was becoming depressed. I knew I could not take on any more health issues. I did not want the world to see me suffer, yet I could not deal with all of these continued, mixed emotions any longer. Finally, in early 2014, at one of my weekly visits to the doctor, I sat and cried. My doctor was terrific. He just listened. After I described how I was feeling, he prescribed a small dosage of antidepressants. Yes, I was hesitant because the stigma of taking antidepressants; I was being told I was depressed on top of everything else! I was on so many other medications and supplements, I did not want to add one more medication to my list. However, I did not feel I had a choice. I really was slowly losing my mind! I took the medication for about six months, and it was helpful. However, my health still was not 100 percent. I was still taking multiple medications, still having multiple symptoms, and still depressed.

My manager, who was also a good friend, would continuously ask about my health and noticed I was not myself. After speaking with him about my frustrations, he said I needed to be my own health advocate. Instead of relying on the doctors and their recommendations, I needed to question the doctors, the diagnoses, and the suggested treatments. This made sense. Why had I not been challenging the doctors? Why had I not been researching more of my issues or questioning the treatment and medications I had been prescribed? The biggest reason was time! I had a full-time job, I had two young kids, I had a husband who traveled for work, and I wanted a normal life!

After realizing I needed to take his advice and become my own health advocate, I opted to take a leave of absence from my job. With the support of my family and my manager, I took four weeks off. I was able to schedule appointments with multiple practitioners and have time to research the diagnoses, the treatments, and the side effects. I was taking my health into my own hands. Unfortunately, during this time off, it became apparent that the doctors maybe did not know all the answers (*more on that later*) to my health issues. I had to find a solution myself.

One morning during my leave, I Googled "how to heal myself." The Institute of Integrative Nutrition (IIN)[10] came up on the search. IIN was an online school that focused on health and nutrition. It suggested that through nutrition, one could learn to heal oneself. Because I was working full time, I did not think this was really an option. I was already too busy. I could not add online classes for one whole year on top of my schedule. In addition, the classes were not free. After a few days of contemplation, I knew I needed to do something other than spend more time at doctor's offices. I took a leap of faith. *This school may be my answer to restoring my health.* I could learn to heal myself. I

---

10 www.Integrativenutrition.com

would be my own health advocate. And the greatest bonus—I could meet other people and get the support I had been continuously seeking.

What I learned at IIN was priceless and life changing. I learned how to determine what worked best for me. I learned that everyone is different and that solutions may change over time. While one solution worked for me for a few months, I may need to experiment with other suggestions. I learned to experiment with different foods, activities, and self-care regimens to try to heal myself. I began to understand how my body reacted to certain foods. Ultimately, I was able to eliminate all medications entirely. Yes, this was simply amazing!

The biggest educational value was learning and experimenting with different nutritional theories. By changing my diet as I learned about different nutritional theories, I began to understand my body and how it reacted to different foods. I began to see that not all diets were equal. A person having great success with one diet may not work for me. I started to experiment with many dietary theories. The first diet was to attempt a vegan lifestyle. This meant no animal by-products, no meat, no eggs, and no dairy—it was strictly plant based.[11] The vegan lifestyle was certainly difficult to embrace. *I had to give up meat?* I grew up in the Midwest, where steak and potatoes were prepared for dinner every night. I tried the vegan lifestyle for about a month and failed miserably. I was hungry all the time despite eating lots of carrots

11 Institute of Integrative Nutrition, Health Coach Training Program May 2014

and other vegetables. I was not feeling full after any meal and started to lack energy on a daily basis. I was tired and exhausted all the time. OK, yes, part of this fatigue could have been my lifestyle. I was working full time, had two daughters involved in numerous activities, and had many doctor appointments, and I was still trying to maintain a reasonable social life.

Without wanting to change my lifestyle, I gave up the vegan attempt and tried the vegetarian lifestyle. Vegetarian was similar to vegan, but I could add animal products like butter, but still no meat or fish.[12] After about a month, I was not sure I could maintain this style of eating. I craved chicken, turkey, and beef. I wanted a form of protein other than beans! Unfortunately, without being able to fully commit to the vegetarian lifestyle, I found the vegetarian diet was also difficult to maintain.

Giving up both vegan and vegetarian diets, I decided to try another dietary plan, which was to remove red meat. This was a good idea until I was diagnosed with adrenal fatigue and iron and blood deficiency. My doctor suggested I add red meat back into my diet to get a large dosage of iron. *OMG! I cannot win!* The dietary changes were exciting at first because I had control of the food I was eating and knew how they affected my body. Now, I felt like I lost all control. I was making a major overhaul of how I was eating on a weekly basis. I was consistently

---

12 Institute of Integrative Nutrition, Health Coach Training Program May 2014

changing my pantry, throwing away foods, and buying new foods and different groceries to adhere to new dietary theories. I was able to manage it because I wanted to be in control of my health. By changing my diet, I was doing just that. Yet, the frustration was building by the continuous changes to my diet without positive results, and now the doctor had said to stop avoiding red meat! *I give up!* Unable to find one dietary theory that worked best, I became depressed again and disheartened because I was trying to eat healthy, but I was not healing. My symptoms were increasing, not decreasing. I was spending the majority of my time just finding foods I could eat, yet the time spent seemed foolish because I was not getting better.

5

Cleansed Mind

Motion brings clarity.

—UNKNOWN

After many dietary changes and building frustration with no results, I had to find another way to heal myself. IIN taught me to look deeper within. I needed to find the cause of my health issues instead of looking only at the effects. I had to look beyond food. The symptoms like weight gain, depression, fatigue, and auto-immune diseases were all the effects of something going on in my life, and I knew food could not heal me if outside factors were also contributing. Things like stress, poor nutrition, overexertion in physical activity, poor relationships, and a stressful career could be the cause of my health problems. I needed to look at the world around me. I could continue to experiment with food, but I could not assume food was the one solution to a healthier me. It could just be my lifestyle choices.

Reviewing my lifestyle did not lead me to any insights at this time. I thought my lifestyle was fine. I had a great job, my kids were active, I worked out every day, and now I was eating healthier. What did I need to change? Well, I did not have much time to ponder my lifestyle because I now had bigger issues. During my leave from work, I mentioned I visited several doctors. I saw an internal-medicine doctor, an endocrinologist, a urologist, an allergist, and a rheumatologist. The results? In May/June of 2014, I was diagnosed with chronic kidney and bladder infections, low stomach acid, food allergies and sensitivities, kidney disease, small-intestinal bacteria overgrowth, irritable bowel syndrome, and leaky gut syndrome. The worst part? They also found a tumor on my liver and a cyst on my kidney. After much panic, the doctors completed more tests and eliminated any concern from the benign tumor on my liver or the cyst on my kidney, yet, one test did come back positive. I had a positive antinuclear antibody (ANA) test result, indicating I could have lupus. *Holy crap!*

To say the least, my leave of absence was more stressful and more emotional than I had ever imagined. More tests were completed because of the ANA positive test result. The tests came back negative. The additional tests did not show anything more, so the doctors were clueless.

At that point, I really thought I was going to lose my mind. I had been to so many doctors practicing traditional and nontraditional medicine, and yet the tests and the results brought no further clarity. I was starting to wonder how else I can deal with the continuing roller coaster I was on. One idea was meditation. Many nontraditional practitioners suggested I meditate to help clear my mind. I had not thought about meditation much up to this time since I was journaling and did not understand the benefits of meditation, nor did I think I had the time. *Honestly, I thought meditation was for the monks.* Don't get me wrong, I would do yoga and sit quietly for a few minutes afterward, but I never really considered that as meditation.

I started to read a little more about meditation and read about many benefits to quieting my mind. Also, as I continued my classes with IIN, a few guest speakers spoke about the benefits of meditation as well. The key takeaway was that by quieting your mind, your mind brings clarity to your thoughts and actions. After more research and more frustration with my doctors, I decided I would try meditation. Side note and funny story (or at least I think so): I remember sitting at work one day, many moons ago, and literally staring at my cube wall for twenty minutes trying to "meditate." It was the most boring thing I had ever done. I recall thinking, *This is dumb and such a waste of valuable time. Who does this stuff?* Despite my earlier experience, I decided to start by intentionally sitting longer after yoga. I told myself I would try to sit for five minutes. To my disbelief, I did, and I eventually worked up to as long as twenty minutes following yoga. After doing this "meditation" a few times, I began to realize I was more patient throughout the day, more content, and just happier. *Who knew?*

After seeing the advantages of meditation after yoga, I began to sit in bed at nights or in a quiet room. I learned a couple techniques through IIN for mindful breathing to help get my mind and body calmed down and relaxed. Several techniques, such as just shutting my eyes and focusing on my breathing or count my breaths in and out (in—one, two, three, four; out—one, two, three, four) were wonderful ways to calm my mind. Having practiced quietly sitting many times, it dawned on me that I may actually be meditating. The benefits I experienced from quieting my mind were astonishing. I was feeling more relaxed and calmer throughout the day. I was seeing a reduction in my stress levels, and I had a greater ability to handle frustrations more effectively.

Having learned about meditation and having practiced it for a couple of weeks, I was gaining a different perspective. I learned that I may not be where I want to be, but that I was doing the best I could *right now*. Yes, I was not feeling 100 percent normal. I was continuously adjusting and readjusting my life with each new diagnosis. I was not able to be as active as I wanted with my kids or spend quality time focusing on my work or my marriage. However, I was still healthier than some people. I was not battling cancer. I had not lost a loved one. I was not living on the streets. I had two healthy children, a good job, and the ability to visit doctors of my choosing. I was healthy enough to still live my life as successfully as I could. As my perspective began to change, I was able to comprehend that everyone struggles with something at some point in time. This was my struggle. Again, I may not be where I want to be, but I'm doing the best I can right now. I had been so busy trying to find out why this was happening to me, I was failing to see the positive changes that journaling, juicing, and now meditation were providing me.

6

All About Me

Do not give up; the beginning is always the hardest.

—FORTUNE COOKIE

With this newfound perspective, I had the motivation to focus on the positive changes and not get stuck in the "why me" syndrome. Several nontraditional doctors said I should find different ways to focus on self-care. They suggested massage, acupuncture, or talk therapy. Running in a thousand different directions with kids, work, marriage, diet, and doctor visits, I personally did not feel I had the time to do any of them. I also did not want to have one more appointment for anything! In additon, the time spent for massage, acupuncture, or talk therapy would take away from my family. I had already devoted so much of my time trying to figure out how to heal myself that taking more time away seemed selfish. *Ugh! How do I take more time for me without feeling guilty?*

Going back to "doing the best I can right now," I brought up the idea of seeking alternative self-care solutions with my family. Everyone thought it was a great idea! *I think because they were getting tired of my sour attitude!* With their enthusiasm, I decided to look for something not related to food, doctors, or diets. I remembered what the practitioners suggested and decided to try massage therapy. Personally, I always thought massage therapy was for sore muscles or just time to relax for an hour. Yes, I had had massages in the past, but I was never a big fan. I was not crazy about people touching me all over my body, no matter what the purpose! Nonetheless, I took a chance and found a massage therapist near me who owned her own small business. The website described the many benefits of massage therapy such as stress relief, relaxation, improved circulation and posture, and a strengthened immune system. [13]

I had no idea massage therapy could promote all of those health benefits. *I needed all the help I could get!* I made an appointment as quickly as I could. The first couple of times were uncomfortable, and my masseuse would constantly talk during the session. *I thought massage therapists were supposed to be silent when giving massages?* Well, to my surprise, I learned so much from her. She taught me about the power of touch through

---

13 www.healingtouchofmassage.com

massage therapy. She could feel when I was stressed, sad, or upset. She could tell if I was not feeling well. I was shocked she could tell so much about me just by massaging my shoulders, arms, or neck!

Another large insight came when I was beginning to feel more relaxed, more loving, and more patient with my family. I once heard that you need twenty physical touches a day to survive. I did not put this together with my family or my life. With all of my health problems, my relationship with my husband was diminishing. We did not have much physical intimacy anymore because of my physical pain and likely because of my focus on my health journey. I had not realized how deprived, lonely, and unloved I felt. This was the first time I realized my marriage was a mess. Unfortunately, I did not know how to change my marriage, so massage therapy was how I obtained my touch. Massage gave me the physical touch I was craving. It became a time for me to relax and heal more than just relieve sore muscles. Because I was getting physically touched, I honestly believe I became more open and loving to my children and my husband. I would have never dreamt in a million years that massage therapy would provide such a benefit to me.

Seeing the benefits of massage therapy, I also wanted to experiment with other self-care options. That's why I sought out acupuncture. I had not heard much about Chinese medicine before, but again, I was open to the possibility of healing through nontraditional medicine.

Acupuncture is inserting tiny needles into pressure points on your body, which in turn trigger organs in the body to respond.[14] *Hmm!* With that in mind, I was not comfortable with just any person inserting needles into my body, so I wanted to find someone with excellent credentials! Referrals led me to a woman in a nearby city. Again, I took a leap of faith and made an appointment. The first visit was long because she asked so many questions about my life, my illnesses, and my day-to-day activities. After speaking with the acupuncturist for what seemed like an hour, she said she could determine what was going on within my body. In my case, she suspected I had adrenal fatigue and blood deficiency. She also said my midsection (abdomen, bladder, liver, kidneys) was heavily stressed and could be failing. She reassured me that acupuncture would help me.

After several visits with her, I was beginning to see some change. I was calmer. I felt more grounded. I was happier. My bladder was changing. I was not experiencing so many infections. The frequent trips to the bathroom were reduced. The bloating within my abdomen was decreasing. I actually thought acupuncture was calming my internal organs. I think it was making me feel lighter from the inside out.

Continuing with acupuncture, I learned how my body was yin and yang and how foods as well as emotions could impact my body.

---

14 http://zenhealingcentermn.com/Services.html

The Chinese believe yin-yang symbols represent perfect balance.[15] For example, yin represents dark, water, and cold, whereas yang represents light, fire, and heat.[16] My acupuncturist explained I had more yang (fire and heat) within my body and how some foods are yin in character and some are yang in character. She recommended different foods to add or remove from my diet based on the yin-yang system. For instance, she suggested I drink stinging nettle or dandelion tea and eat roasted cabbage with olive oil, fennel seeds, and salt and pepper and avoid raw veggies. My acupuncturist often recommended books to read or herbs and supplements to try to help balance my yin and yang. This view into Chinese medicine was quite fascinating, and I was definitely seeing the benefits of this nontraditional form of medicine.

Through massage therapy and acupuncture, I was feeling more like a human being again. I learned about holistic treatments for health issues. I learned that the most important healing technique was to take care of myself. Women tend to put their children and families first and do not spend the same amount of time caring for themselves as they do for others. In my doctor visits, many doctors insisted I had to be healthy in order to care for my family. If I'm not healthy, then my family will suffer. It took many people and many times of hearing this before it sunk in. *I'm stubborn too.*

---

15 http://www.whats-your-sign.com/yin-yang-symbols.html
16 http://www.whats-your-sign.com/yin-yang-symbols.html

With the positive changes I was experiencing with journaling, juicing, massage therapy, and acupuncture, I eventually worked hard to carve out a few minutes each day to do something just for me. I would try to find time each day, even if it was just ten minutes, to read a few pages of a book or magazine, to write a letter to a friend or in my journal, to take my dog for a walk, to call or text a friend, to listen to music in my car, or to just lock the door and sing in the shower. I had not made myself a priority as our lives were constantly moving. Now, I was finally making an effort—yes, I was still guilt-ridden, but I did make an effort to stop and smell the roses. I gathered my family would rather have me spend twenty minutes to myself each day and have a healthy wife, mom, and daughter than have me be sick, sad, unhappy, or maybe absent forever.

7

Gratitude for Love

Never ignore a person who loves you, cares for you, and misses you.
Because one day, you may wake up from your sleep and realize you
lost the moon while counting the stars.

—Unknown

aking more time for myself was eye-opening. I was trying to see the world in a nicer light. I was beginning to see I needed to be thankful for so much in my life. I needed to count my blessings and be thankful for what I had versus looking at what I did not have. Admittedly, though, I was still feeling sorry for myself at times. *Why me? Why can't I get healthy? Why doesn't anyone understand?* Despite my "need to be thankful" attitude, I was not happy with myself or my situation at many points in this journey. Even though I was able to find time to focus on me, I was still very frustrated with my spouse, my friends, and my family. I was taking all these steps to get better, and I had hoped the people in my life would also help me. The sad thing was that they did not—at least not from my point of view. Yes, I was thankful for the people who took time out of their day to help me find recipes or cook a meal or just go for a walk. Yet, my frustration with my health was consuming my mind. I did not understand why I was still sick. I did not understand why so many doctors still could not figure out what was wrong with me.

At one point while I was attending IIN, I listened to a lecture by James Pawelski and he decribed a practice called three blessings.[17] Basically, you are to say three things that happened during the day that you would consider blessings. You should also be able to explain why those things were blessings. The advantage of doing this even for just twenty-one days would be increased happiness and appreciation. *Yes, I did need to be happier and appreciate more.*

Trying to be more thankful, I started writing three blessings in my journal every day. Sometimes I did not have time to write them in my journal, so I would say them outloud to myself before I went to bed. After about two weeks, I started to realize my attitude was changing. I was beginning to see the good things from the day instead of the negative events. Because I was experiencing a positive result, I wanted to include the whole family. I thought this would be a great practice to

---

17 Institute of Integrative Nutrition, Health Coach Training Program May 2014

start with the kids, so they could also see the positive things in life and appreciate the little things instead of always expecting more. When I made the suggestion, everyone was happy to give it a try.

Generally, before bedtime, we would sit together and all share three positive things or three blessings that happened during the day. I would generally go first to provide examples of actions, events, or things people did or said that were blessings to me. After the kids said their blessings, I would ask why they were blessings. The most popular answer was because they were! *Pick your battles, right?* Some days, the three blessings were just that school was fun or there was a good call at work. Other times, we were thankful for the time with grandparents or with friends, a new treatment plan, or just time for a bike ride. The entire family found the three blessings were not difficult to think of, and it was not time consuming. We were just taking a small bit of time to remember the good things in the day! And yes, this practice was making my girls happier and more grateful for everything they did and had. Instead of complaining about something that happened or did not happen, they were beginning to focus on the positive aspects of the day.

As we continued expressing our blessings, I heard about another idea for showing gratitude that entailed writing ten gratitude statements daily.[18] Yes, it's as easy as it sounds. I was to write ten things I was

18 Institute of Integrative Nutrition, Health Coach Training Program May 2014

grateful for that day. So, in addition to the three blessings, I would also write ten positive things from the day. Again, having limited time, I would sometimes have to write ten gratitude statements in anticipation of the day if I could carve out some time in the morning. I would write things, such as *I'm grateful for the sun shining in the car this morning on my way to work, I'm grateful for the compliment on my shirt I received from a stranger, I'm grateful for two healthy children,* or *I'm grateful my husband put the dishes away today.* It's the small things, right?

I found that this practice of writing ten positive statements encouraged me to change my outlook. I began to think more positively versus viewing everything from a negative viewpoint. This also helped me realize how many wonderful people I had in my life. I had many things to be grateful for. I had a successful career, income to pay for medical expenses not covered by insurance *(there were many)*, time away from work to attend doctor appointments, treatments for my various diagnoses, and caring people around me. I truly had many things to be thankful for on a daily basis. By writing ten gratitude statements, I was able to turn my bad moods into better moods. I found I began to look for the good in the day or start the day on a positive note instead of complaining.

An inspiring example of being more grateful is the story about Geneen Roth.[19] At a live conference in New York this past spring, Geneen Roth spoke about how she had lost all her money, savings, and

19 www.geneenroth.com

investments and was still able to be grateful for what she had. [20] I can't do the story justice, but she explained how she received a phone call and was told all of their money, their savings, and their investments were lost. Everything, she and her husband had worked so hard for was gone. They fell victim to the Bernie Madoff scandal. Geneen Roth said that she immediately called her husband, who was out of town, and cried. After gathering herself, she said she then sat down and counted all the things she still had, like a roof over her head, clothes on her back, good health, and supportive friends. I don't know about you, but I'm pretty sure my first reaction would have been sheer panic! I was truly inspired by Geneen Roth. I was in awe at how one person could lose all of her wealth in one day and still have the grace and the patience to focus on the positive things in life. *Amazing!* Here I was, moping around because of health issues, yet I still had all my money, investments, and savings. This inspired me to appreciate the things I did have!

Finally, with having learned about and done these many different practices for being grateful, I understood I needed to focus on the good, not the bad. I needed to be grateful there were doctors in my city that could and were willing to help me. I needed to be grateful for the people who did offer support. I needed to quit feeling sorry for myself!

---

20 April 2015 Integrative Nutrition Live Conference

8

Broken Home

Sometimes when things are falling apart,

they may actually be falling into place.

—U<small>NKNOWN</small>

While I did become more grateful, my body was still not healing. I was still struggling with symptoms like muscle loss, severe fatigue, severe bloating, inflammation, acne, weight gain, and increasingly more food allergies or sensitivities. I began to wonder what was really going on in my body. Through IIN, I learned about symptoms and cause and effect. I had tried to look at my lifestyle previously in order to determine if my lifestyle may be a cause of my health issues, but I did not see any changes I needed to make at that time.

While it seemed I was doing all the right things for my health, I needed to look beyond food and self-care. I needed to indeed look at my lifestyle and my relationships. Maybe my lifestyle was causing increased stress and/or frustration. The changes I was making to my food, my self-care, and my devotion to healthy living were working, but it was not enough. When I began to look inward, I did see my relationships were impacted. I had not noticed this earlier because I was so focused on trying to get better and get healthier. I began to realize how many of my relationships were actually impacted. Even though I was focusing on many positive aspects of my health and life, I was still feeling lost and alone—now more than ever before. I was feeling as if nobody cared.

Understand, I was not sharing my story with everyone (except via my blog) because many people, friends and family, were critical of my attitude. I would often hear, "You don't look sick" or "You are always so happy." Yes, I did not look sick because everything wrong was internal. I was trying to be positive and happy because it was easier to smile and not talk about my problems than have to explain my most recent diagnosis or treatment. *Nobody wants to hear that!* Because I was feeling unsupported and misunderstood, I began to limit my communications with others and withdraw from friends and family. I avoided social gatherings. If I did go, I would hang back from the crowd or conversation. Honestly, my own health was overwhelming for me; how could I expect anyone else to understand? I also did not want people's sympathy. I really wanted their support and under-standing. I wanted someone to give me a hug and say, "Everything will be OK." I wanted someone to offer a shoulder to cry on or act as the pillar of strength I so much needed. I needed someone to push me to keep going.

Aside from my friendships, my health journey was also damag-ing and destroying my marriage. My husband and I had been mar-ried thirteen years, and we spent most of our time together. We often ran errands together and worked on daily chores around the house together. We were a team! We traveled every year with our daughters. We had a very fun, loving relationship. However, after I had the hys-terectomy, we started having a few disagreements, although nothing out of the ordinary. A few months after my bladder surgery was when our relationship took a turn for the worse. I started spending my time finding doctors and attending doctor appointments. I was spending the majority of my time trying to figure out what was wrong with my health and what I could do to fix it. I was (and still am) a very inde-pendent person, so I often did all of this on my own. My husband did not understand the extent of the support I needed or craved. The more I withdrew from our friends, the harder he fought to maintain the relationship with our friends. The problem was that I was viewing this as a rejection. It appeared to me he was picking our friends over my health. It appeared he wanted to spend time with our friends instead of helping or supporting me.

We eventually recognized our struggling relationship and sought marriage counseling. The counseling was helpful for a period of time, but we found our behavior would go back to what brought us to counseling: mistrust, avoidance, and betrayal. Over the course of the two years following my bladder surgery, we had lost our connection. We began to live separate lives. Many times, it felt like we were roommates instead of husband and wife. We lost touch with what a husband and a wife were or should be to each other. In spite of our efforts, marriage counseling was not able to repair our lost connection. Counseling was not changing our relationship permanently. After continuing down the road of failed attempts, we both began to feel unloved and unwanted. I wanted him to support me with my health issues. He wanted me to quit focusing on my health issues. It was a vicious cycle.

In mid-2014, we separated. I wanted to live apart because I felt it was easier to live without him then to deal with my health problems and his problem of being supportive. I did not want to deal with his tactics of trying to persuade me to go out or spend time with people when I preferred to exclude myself. I did not want to fight with him about my dietary restrictions. I did not want to have to deal with his constant bickering about my time going to doctor appointments or my various attempts at different diets. I wanted to focus on me and only me. I wanted to be healthy! I decided I could not be healthy with him so I was better without him. Within six months of the separation, I began the divorce process.

Because I was concerned about how a divorce would impact our then ten-year-old and six-year-old daugthers, I wanted to make the divorce process as painless as possible. While attending a local woman's divorce group, I was introduced to a mediator who indicated mediation was a great route for divorce because it works through the division of assets and the divorce process and teaches each spouse how to communicate with each other before and after the divorce.

As we worked with the mediator, she wanted us to develop personal goals. His goal was to stay married. My goal, again, was to get a divorce. Seeing we were on separate ends of the spectrum, our mediator knew she had her work cut out for her. Her first target was communication. We had to learn to communicate with each other in order to work through our different goals, opinions, and expectations.

The first thing she had us do was communicate our expectations with each other. What did I expect from myself through this mediation process and possible divorce? What did he expect of himself through this mediation process and possible divorce? We were not to communicate what we expected of the other person, only what we expected of ourselves. *Hmm, that's a different approach! Should I not be telling him what I needed to feel supported?* Through this new communication process, we started to learn how to communicate. We learned how to tell the other person exactly what we needed. We learned not to assume the other person already knew. Just because we were married did not mean we can read each other's minds. Having to communicate our expectations of ourselves, we began to work on ourselves. We learned we couldn't change the other person. We could only change ourselves.

This new process was beginning to change my perspective and my attitude. The turning point for me was when the mediator said to me, "Lori, what happens if you are divorced and still sick? What if the divorce doesn't make you better?" Well, I had not thought of that before. I had assumed his lack of support was causing me to be sicker. I was adamant that my health would change by getting a divorce. The mediator mentioned Christian would still be a part of my life, regardless if we were married or not.

She also pointed out how devoted Christian was to me. She commented that she did not know many people, if any, who would stick by my side after I had asked him or her to leave and constantly told him or her all the things he or she has done wrong. *Wow, everything she was saying was true.* I would still have to communicate with Christian because we had two children together. I may still have health problems even after a divorce. Maybe he really did love me even though I had spent the majority of my time on my health and belittling him for things I wanted him to do or do better.

Because of my negative mind-set toward our marriage, I did start, unwillingly at first, to look at *what* he was doing, not *how* he was doing it. We had the same end goal with my health, our kids, and our family, but we were not doing things the same way to reach the same end goals. Either one of our ways was good, but I was focusing only on my way. I had to start to appreciate him for the good things done: "Thanks for doing the dishes" instead of "You didn't put them away in the right spot." "Thanks for taking out the garbage" instead of "You didn't take it out sooner." I was beginning to understand how my illness affected him.

In addition to my change of attitude, Christian was now more willing to listen to and understand ways he could support me. He also learned he had a few things to work on too. *See, it's not all about me!* For starters, he had to deal with accountability. He would always tell me he would help me, but he failed on the execution. I would come home from a doctor's appointment and explain what I needed to do. He would say he would do whatever he could, but when it came time to make changes to our lifestyle or diet or our relationship, he would back down. I was left to do it myself, to defend myself, to constantly explain myself. With mediation, he now had someone other than me to hold him accountable. We were now paying someone else to ensure he followed through with what he said he would do. *Maybe a hit to the pocketbook would actually help!*

With the change in both of our attitudes, I slowly came around to my marriage. We were learning how to show compassion for each other. We were learning to ask why each other did something instead of criticizing what the other person did. We were trying to understand the other person's point of view and look at each situation with empathy instead of anger and frustration. We were learning to appreciate we were doing the best we could.

9

Gotta Have Faith

Be gentle with yourself; you are doing the best you can.

—Unknown

As I changed my thinking and my attitude, I was still not without major lows. At one point after I started the divorce process and continued to withdraw from my friends and family, I eventually hit rock bottom. I could not figure out how to deal with my failing marriage, my failing health, my unsupportive friends or family, and my stressful career. I was willing to end my marriage. I was willing to avoid my friends. I was willing to withdraw from my family especially since they were upset with my decision to file for divorce. I would have rather spent long and stressful hours at my job than take time to repair my marriage or friendships. I did not have time to prepare foods to eat the way I was being told to eat. I did not have time to go to different doctor appointments or to continue to go to massage therapy and acupuncture. The icing on the cake was when I was diagnosed with Raynaud's phenomenon and candida, which entailed more dietary restrictions and more tests. With work, divorce, and now more health issues, I was beyond exhausted, beyond frustrated, and beyond help!

In March 2015, I sat in my office and prayed. I prayed God would send an angel to help. I was at rock bottom. I sat in my home office and cried. I was broken. I needed someone—anyone—to help me. At the time, I did not feel I had my family, my friends, or my husband to help me. I prayed God would send an angel because I was not going to survive another day. *I cannot do any more. Period.*

Within hours of my prayer, my husband asked if he could take me on a trip even though we were separated. He knew I was struggling and wanted to help me despite our circumstances. I reluctantly agreed. I later learned this may be the miracle I prayed for. We went away for a week without kids, without work, and without stress. I read. I walked. We talked. We had a great time. After noticing how much better I felt after this trip, we decided to take the girls on a spring break trip. We again had a great time!

On the way home from our second trip, I started reading *You Can, You Will* by Joel Osteen.[21] I could not put the book down the entire plane ride home. This book reinforced that I needed to change my thinking and my perspective on my marriage and on my health. The

---

21 https://www.joelosteen.com/Pages/youcanyouwill.aspx

book provided options to start speaking more positively every day and focus on the good versus always seeing the bad. While this was something I thought I was already doing, this book reinforced and improved it. I do want to improve myself. I do want to be a better person.

After reading the book and incorporating some positive affirmations in my daily life for a few weeks, I eventually pieced it together that other things in my life were affecting my health negatively, not necessarily just my marriage. I began to see how work was stressful and the 100 percent focus on my diet and dietary restrictions were stressful. This stress was ruining my relationships, my marriage, my health, and ultimately…me.

These healthy habits began to finally and permanently change my perspective on my marriage, my health, and my relationships. Many facets in my life became positively impacted. First, my family began to eat healthier to help support me. They tried to eat whole, natural foods and tried to reduce processed sugar. My youngest daughter started reading sugar labels at only seven years old. At one time, she threw away a bottle of soda because she said it contained too much sugar and asked what healthier options existed. Wow, I was so impressed! As a family, we also decided to avoid sugar for three days, and Brityn asked if we could try it again for four days the following next week. I couldn't have been prouder!

In addition, my oldest daughter Ella started baking foods with ingredients I could eat (and those which were healthier options). She would modify recipes to include ingredients I could eat and started to experiment with different cakes and cookies. On several occasions, she would say her goal was to create and own her own gluten-free, dairy-free, and nut-free bakery. *Yes, you can!*

Another positive impact on my life was new and stronger friendships. I developed amazing friendships with two women from IIN. I also met a wonderful woman through a woman's divorce group. All three of these women were and continue to be inspirations to me on a daily basis! In addition, I also learned to cherish my old friendships. I learned to appreciate the support my friends gave me in different ways, like helping me cook meals, experimenting with new foods, and trying new restaurants as well as just checking in with me on a daily or weekly basis.

The most profound impact was experiencing unconditional love from my husband and a couple dear friends. They all were nonjudgmental. They never walked away in the midst of my good or bad decisions. They let me make decisions and always stood beside me in case I needed them without judging or wavering. And most of all, they celebrated my successes no matter how big or small. I was not able to see this devotion and love before. *Thank you!*

10

Love or Money

How will you know it's the right decision if you never make it?

—Unknown

My life was changing. I was starting to see the positive things in my life instead of dwelling on the negative health issues and the problems in my marriage. With this new outlook on life, I started to realize my job was extremely stressful. I worked long hours. *Could my job be contributing to my continuing health issues?* Honestly, I loved my job. I had great flexibility. I was climbing the corporate ladder. Yet, as I built a stronger relationship with my husband and recognized the added stress from my job, we contemplated whether I should leave it. I had been in the legal profession for thirteen years, working within the technology area the last four. I knew from my leave of absence in May 2014 that my manager would be supportive.

When I had said I needed to take a leave of absence in 2014, he said to just go; we've got you covered. He lightened my workload when I returned and continuously asked what he could do to help me both personally or professionally.

I also found I had a new passion for health and wellness. I wanted to help others who were going through similar circumstances and help them regain their health. I wanted to inspire people. I wanted someone to look at me and say, "Because of you, I didn't give up." I was always told that I have a tender heart and compassion for others, so maybe I should try something to help others. I learned through IIN that by helping others, I would also be helping myself. *Is this something I could really do?*

In May of 2015, after much prayer, I finally made the decision to leave my job. I knew my marriage was regaining ground. I realized I had wonderful, supportive friends, and my family was beginning to come around to the positive changes I was making. Making this decision was difficult and scary. My husband and I sat down and looked at our finances to ensure we had financial security. I was giving up a monstrous career, large income, and flexibility to work from home along with a great network of people. I enlisted support from family and prayed for new direction and new opportunities.

I cannot begin to tell you how this decision changed my life. I felt happier, healthier, and freer than I ever had throughout this health journey. I had such peace with this decision. I looked back at many decisions I made throughout the last five years and realized I had never felt this content. Yes, I was giving up a hefty salary and continued career growth. However, I felt a new chapter was opening for me. I would be able to pursue my dreams. My health journey had given me the courage, the confidence, and the motivation to be better, to do better, and to help make other people's lives better.

11

All Powered Up

I love the person I've become because I fought to become her.

—KACI DIANE

ooking back, I now know how lost in health I was. I look at the decisions I made, whether they were good or bad, and understand I could, and maybe should have, made different decisions through my health journey. However, I appreciate the decisions made me who I am today. I am stronger. I am wiser. I am healthier.

Most importantly, I learned so many wonderful things. I learned about journaling, juicing, meditation, massage therapy, and acupuncture. I learned to create time and space for my healing whether it be from broken relationships or continued health diagnoses. I learned to be grateful and focus on the positive aspects of my life and concentrate on what is going well. I gained a renewed faith in God and the power of daily affirmations. I learned outside factors like career and relationships contribute to health and illness. I learned through proper care, attention, and maintenance, I could overcome my health challenges.

I also have a greater awareness to be my own health advocate. I need to take the time to research doctors, diagnoses, suggested treatments, and prescriptions. It is OK to ask doctors questions, to ask for references, to ask for statistics, and to ask about side effects. It is OK to challenge doctors and seek second, third, or fourth opinions. That is how we will improve our health care system and improve our own health. That is how I will improve my health.

I cannot imagine my life differently than it is today. So many lessons learned and so many new beginnings. I am blessed to have so much and now have the clarity to see it. I have gained healthier and happier relationships with friends, family, and my husband. Through the wonderful education at IIN, sacrifice, tears, pain, and struggle, I have a renewed appreciation for friends and family and am rebuilding my marriage. I know because of this journey and the lessons I have learned that my health will eventually improve. *No, it is not perfect yet!* I may not be where I want to be, but I'm doing the best I can RIGHT NOW.

One of my favorite quotes is, "You never know how strong you are until being strong is the only choice you have."[22] I was lost in health

22 Unknown

but through the love of many, I forged ahead, even at times when I did not think I would survive another day. Through failures, successes and prayers, I learned how to change my life and my health. I would not trade my journey for the world, because what I gained on my journey, has given me a new world!

www.ingramcontent.com/pod-product-compliance
Lightning Source LLC
Chambersburg PA
CBHW070319290526
45791CB00003B/1174